10-MINUTE BALANCE WORKOUTS FOR SENIORS

Simple Illustrated Exercises Elderly of Any Level Can Do at Home to Drastically Improve Balance, Build Strength, and Prevent Fall-Related Injuries

Steve Donovan

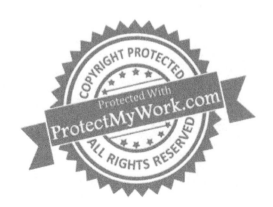

TABLE OF CONTENTS

INTRODUCTION

You'll never have to worry about falling. Do you think this is a startling opening comment? It isn't really, as it is a fact of life that as you get older you are more prone to falls, which could have serious consequences. Once you understand why you are prone to falling, you can address the issues. This book is going to help you achieve much more stability than you have at the moment.

When you were a baby, falling was part of your development. You did not have control of much of your body. Everything had to be learnt, partly by family encouragement and partly by the desire to emulate everyone else. Apart from scooting around on the floor, you yearned to balance well enough to take those first tottery steps. You learned how to control all aspects of your body so that they could work together to stand up and take those first steps. Balance was important to you then, and stayed important as you got older. As you progress through life, you no longer have to spend time figuring out how to stay upright. You get on with living–and maybe you will trip, but you will seldom fall. And if you do fall, you can manage to, pick yourself up, dust yourself off, and start all over again (as sang in the song, "Pick Yourself Up," by Fred Astaire). Usually, the only damage that will be done is damage to your self-esteem; but once embarrassment wears off, you will be fine.

As you get older, life tends to become a bit more sedentary and aches and pains become more common; and if you don't watch yourself, your muscles will become weaker and falling will become a very real hazard. Weak muscles encourage falling; and with weak muscles, you are going to battle to get up without help. Falling is a very real threat for the sedentary elderly. It is a horrible fact that your bones break more easily when you are old, and recovery from broken bones is longer and more fraught with danger than with younger people. Some elderly folks never recover from a broken bone, particularly if it is in the legs or hips.

So seniors—get up and get active. You have taken the first step by buying this book. Your next step is to use it to get the best out of your senior years. Fit seniors have the world to enjoy.

THE GOALS OF THIS BOOK

This book aims to help sedentary seniors gain strength in their limbs—particularly their lower limbs. If your legs are strong, you are less likely to fall—but if you do fall, you will have the strength in your legs to get up with little or no help. You will probably need to grab on to something to help you up, so this book will also cover strengthening of the arms and upper body.

This book will help you understand why falling is more prevalent in the elderly, and it will give you tips on how you can stay more stable on your feet.

The exercises are fun and easy to do, and they don't take much time. They are graded to suit your level of fitness. The secret is to get a good routine going. Once a week will not cut it. The ideal pattern is 10 minutes per day, every day—or at least 3 times per week once you get fit.

You do not need much equipment. The most basic need is a sturdy chair. You will be using the chair for seated exercises and also to help you maintain your balance for the standing exercises. As you get fitter, you may want to introduce resistance bands and weights. Just a quick tip about weights—use water bottles filled with water. You can adjust the water level (or bottle size) to suit your current fitness level. And those two bottles will have been recycled and put to good use!

DETAILING THE STRUCTURE OF THIS BOOK

CHAPTER 1: THE IMPORTANCE OF BALANCE

This chapter deals with the physiological reasons of why the loss of balance occurs. It gets a bit technical, but it will help you understand why balance is important and why we become slightly physically imbalanced as we age. Age and illness play a big part in maintaining balance. If you battle to stay balanced, it is no shame to consider using a walking aid. And just a note: Some of the standing and walking exercises can be adjusted for those who use walkers.

CHAPTER 2: BALANCE TESTS

You can't improve your future balance if you don't know your current condition. Several tests will be discussed. I suggest you make a note of your results and repeat the tests after a few sessions, and then maybe once a month thereafter.

CHAPTER 3: VESTIBULAR REHABILITATION EXERCISES

This is the easiest and most friendly way to start working on balance and dizziness. There is a section in Chapter 1 that explains how the vestibular system causes dizziness and imbalance. Illness or age can result in damage to the vestibular system. The exercises in this chapter will help you regain balance, as long as there is no permanent damage. If there is permanent damage, it is still not a concern. Our brain is a wonderful organ, and it will adjust to help you maintain your balance. This is called vestibular compensation.

CHAPTER 4: SEATED BALANCE WORKOUTS

After vestibular rehab, seated exercises are the easiest to perform for beginners.

If you are a beginner or are wheelchair bound or rely heavily on a walking aid, these exercises are for you. They will help you strengthen your limbs, as well as your core muscles. Your core is important in maintaining balance. There have been instances where reliance on equipment has diminished once the core is strengthened. Also, standing balance will improve.

CHAPTER 5: CORE STRENGTH WORKOUT

This chapter deals solely with core strengthening. Core strength is essential to ensure great stability and to support a person's weight, so it must be a priority.

CHAPTER 6: STANDING BALANCE WORKOUT—BEGINNER

After having improved your balance with the past workouts, you can step up and perform standing balance exercises.

Some of these exercises can be adapted for use with a walking aid. A chair will be useful to help you maintain your balance. If you are holding on with both hands, make sure that you do not lean on the chair. It is preferable to just use a light touch when needed.

CHAPTER 7: STANDING BALANCE WORKOUT—INTERMEDIATE

Step up time again... This chapter will include more advanced exercises and is a continuation from Chapter 6.

CHAPTER 8: STANDING BALANCE WORKOUT—ADVANCED

When the exercises in the previous section seem to be easy, it is time to step up once again and move through the exercises in this chapter.

Chapter 9: Full-Body Strength Workout

Balance and strength are related, hence the importance of strength exercises for preventing bad falls.

You may find some of these challenging, but do the best you can. As the sessions progress, you will find these easier. Your balance and core strength will improve.

Chapter 10: 6-Week Training Plan

Following a smart, well-structured training plan is essential to build balance in the quickest and safest way.

If you need assistance with how long to stay on any of the given plans, this chapter will help, as it takes you through a 6-week program. Of course, you can spend a bit more time on each phase if you feel you need it.

Chapter 11: Alphabetical Index

If you want to find your favorite exercises, a quick indicator of the chapter in which they are included can be found here.

Conclusion

This is a brief summary of what the book covered and a friendly reminder to not procrastinate and start the week plan now.

HOW DO YOU GET GOOD, QUICK RESULTS?

Practice, practice, practice. Exercise, exercise, exercise!

Unfortunately, there is no quick fix—but if you follow our plan, after a few sessions, you should start to feel some benefits. Anyone can find 10 minutes in a day to devote to their well-being. You need to develop the habit. Set yourself a task to snatch 10 minutes per day to perform these exercises. It will be easier if you set aside a similar time each day. It is said that you can build a habit in 9 days; however, some practitioners say it could take more than 200 days. Now that sounds horribly disheartening. Personally, I have found that it takes me about 3 weeks to develop (or break) a habit. So, perseverance becomes the name of the game.

Your best results will come from these pointers:

- Mindfully perform the exercises. Think about what you are doing. Imagine your success once you have developed the habit of exercising. Don't compile shopping lists, watch TV, or read. Concentrate on what your body is doing. As your brain takes in the techniques, you can relax your concentration a bit.

- Exercise at least three times a week. Every day is preferable, though, particularly in the early stages when you are trying to develop your exercise habit.

- Do the best you can during each session. Some sessions will be easier than others at first. Do not get discouraged.

- Start each session with breathing exercises.

- Shake your limbs out after each exercise.

BREATHING EXERCISES

Sit relaxed in your chair with eyes closed before you perform these exercises:

- Breathe in as deeply as you can, and immediately expel the air with force. Try to empty the lungs, and repeat this 3 times.

- Breathe in for 3, hold for 3, exhale for 3. Repeat this 3 times.

- Breathe in for 4 and control your breath as you breathe out for 10. Repeat this 3 times.

According to Confucius, if you carry away enough stones every day, you can move a mountain ("A Quote From," n.d.). The same applies to exercising. If at first you can't do 10 repetitions or 3 sets, do as many as you can–and tomorrow you may be able to do one more. If you can't hold a balance stance for 10 seconds, hold it for as long as you can. Tomorrow you will hold it for 1 second longer. The exercise mountain will be achieved with perseverance. Do the best you can, and the results will be as quick and as good as you could wish.

EQUIPMENT NEEDED

All you need is a sturdy chair, preferably one with arms—although some exercises will be easier if there are no arms. As the exercises get easier, you may wish to introduce resistance bands or weights. This is entirely up to you. If you use a walking aid, these could be incorporated into the walking exercises.

Make sure your clothes are comfortable. I prefer to exercise in slightly baggy clothes. Shoes are optional, but beginners will balance better if they wear comfortable, sturdy shoes like walking shoes.

As you get better at the exercises, try to do them barefoot or standing on a foam cushion. You will find that other muscles come into play when you change your base.

Chapter 1

THE IMPORTANCE OF BALANCE

Balance is the most critical aspect when it comes to avoiding falling. Unfortunately, many things can upset balance; so it is necessary that we understand the factors disturbing balance, as well as how to combat it (or at least handle it) so that it doesn't become a problem in our daily lives.

We can consider an imaginary line that passes from our head to our toes going through the middle of our body. If our eyes waver off this midline, we may experience imbalance. You may be standing quite still, but when you move your eyes too rapidly to the side, it could set off feelings of nausea and dizziness. If you shake your head from side to side or nod it up and down, your central balance may be disturbed. If someone calls you and you turn your head too fast in their direction, don't be surprised if you become imbalanced. This could lead to a fall, which is bad news for senior citizens.

The center of balance is found in the core. If you have no idea what the core is, imagine one of those men who are ultra-fit with rippling muscles. When you look at the 6-pack, you have found the central part of the core. The core establishes our center of gravity. Any movement that changes that center of gravity could lead to imbalance. A strong core will help prevent balance issues, so many exercises will be focused on strengthening the core.

When you stand relaxed, your feet will usually be slightly apart. This helps us establish a wide base for our body. If you move the feet together, the base becomes smaller, and imbalance can occur.

To maintain balance, we will often compromise by swaying slightly from side to side or by using our arms to help us balance.

When you stand on one leg, your arms and body will move to counteract any swaying that may come from being imbalanced. One of the reasons you become imbalanced is because you have reduced your support base. But balance does not rest entirely on core strength or fluctuations around your support base. Your surroundings could also have an impact—for example, an uneven surface.

Many body parts come into play, and balance can be disrupted by any sudden movements or changes in posture.

When you bend down, you cause many bodily reactions that could upset your balance:

- Your head has been repositioned.

- Your eyes have moved from looking straight ahead.

- You have disturbed your center of gravity.

As you get older, normal wear and tear occurs. You need glasses, and getting used to something like bifocals could cause balance problems. The body parts controlling balance react slower, so you are more prone to overbalance and falling becomes a reality.

The following sections deal with the body parts that affect your balance.

BALANCE AND THE BRAIN

There is no doubt that balance cannot be ignored as you age; maintaining it is crucial—in both mind and body. Strengthening your body through physical activity and specific exercises can help you maintain balance and avoid falls. However, your brain also plays a big role. Having a sharp mind makes it easier to think, as well as remain agile. Word games and Sudoku can help keep the mind active.

The brain is crucial to good balance, and it can be trained to curb imbalance. The only time it will stop helping to maintain balance is if you are ill or stressed. Meditation can help you control stressors in your life.

SENSORY INPUT

In order for you to stay balanced, information is received from three different sources: your eyes, your muscles, and your vestibular organs. All three sources send signals to the brain via nerve impulses sent from sensory receptors.

INPUT FROM YOUR EYES

The retina contains sensory receptors called rods and cones. Low-light conditions are better suited to rods. Cones help us see color, allowing us to see more of the world. As light hits the rods and cones, the brain receives impulses that aid in orienting you in relation to other objects. For example, when you take a stroll in the city, everything lines up vertically, and buildings move in and out of your peripheral vision.

INPUT FROM YOUR MUSCLES

The proprioceptive system of the skin, muscles, and joints consists of sensory receptors responsive to changes in tension or pressure between tissues. For example, your feet feel more pressure in the back when you lean backward. Any time you move your legs, arms, and other parts of your body, sensory receptors send signals to your brain. Together with other information, these tension and pressure signals help you determine your location relative to space.

Sensory impulses from the neck and ankles are of particular importance. Proprioceptive cues on your neck tell you which way your head is turning. Ankle cues indicate your movements or sway in relation to the ground you're standing on and the condition of that surface.

INTEGRATION OF SENSORY INPUT

Information about balance from peripheral sensory organs—eyes, muscles, and joints—is transmitted to your brain stem. It is then combined with knowledge learned from the cerebellum and the cerebral cortex. The cerebellum controls coordination, and the cerebral cortex controls thinking and memory.

In the cerebellum, information is stored about automatic movements acquired from practice. For example, by repeatedly practicing footwork, a soccer player improves the ability to control balance while performing the movement. He builds up muscle memory. The cerebral cortex provides the memory of previous experiences; for example, because snow-covered sidewalks are slick, you are forced to walk differently to avoid slipping on them.

PROCESSING OF CONFLICTING SENSORY INPUT

You can become dizzy if the sensory input coming from your eyes and muscles conflict in some way with each other. For example, this might happen when someone stands next to a large truck that is driving away from the curb. Seeing the truck may give the illusion that they are in motion instead of the truck. Meanwhile, the information from their muscles suggests they aren't moving. In addition, cognitive abilities and memory may cause them to glance away from the moving truck. This is in order to verify that their body has not shifted relative to the ground.

DIZZINESS AND THE VESTIBULAR SYSTEM

You have small sensory receptors in your inner ear called the vestibular system, which is also responsible for maintaining balance. Practically speaking, by looking upward, downward, or sideways, the ear fluid moves within the cavities and channels of the organ. Sensors in your hair cells pick up these changes, and your brain uses this feedback to determine where you are relative to space and your movement. Your body relies on this input to stay in equilibrium and in proper balance.

Dizziness and imbalance are common health concerns for aging adults, as they increase the risk of falling. Despite the fact that the causes of dizziness in seniors are complex, peripheral vestibular dysfunction is a common cause. Benign paroxysmal positional vertigo accounts for the majority of vestibular dysfunction in the elderly, followed by Meniere's disease (a condition of the inner ear characterized by dizziness and loss of hearing).

Every factor involved in the maintenance of balance declines with aging. Age-related declines in peripheral vestibular function are evident from testing of the vestibulo-ocular reflex and the vestibulo-collic reflex. The decline of vestibular function correlates with an age-associated reduction in the number of inner ear hair cells and neurons. It is still a mystery as to what exactly causes cellular degeneration in the inner ear, but it is likely that oxidative damage and genetics have a significant impact (Iwasaki & Yamasoba, 2015).

BAD BALANCE AND FALLS

What makes falls and preventing them so necessary? Let's examine the individual and societal costs of falls.

It is estimated that approximately 8 million Americans of all ages suffer from balance disorders each year. About 25% of people over the age of 65 report having balance problems or needing assistance or equipment in order to walk. There is a substantial spike in the numbers after age 75. It is stated that 4 out of 10 senior citizens will most likely suffer from imbalance ("Basic Facts About," n.d.).

SENIORS AND THE IMPORTANCE OF AVOIDING FALLS

When you are over the age of 65, you are more likely to fall because of balance problems. About one-third of adults in this age bracket, and more than half of those over 75, suffer a fall every year. Women and men are equally impacted.

The dizziness you feel may last for a few minutes or persist for days, months, or a lot longer. Regardless of the reason or duration, it will be challenging for you to keep an upright position for as long as it lasts. There is a possibility that you will have difficulty performing everyday tasks such as showering, getting dressed, preparing food, or moving around the house.

CONSEQUENCES AND TIPS ON HOW TO PREVENT FALLS

It is important that you address your balance problems—not only because falls are a risk, but also because the anxiety associated with falling can lead you to limit your physical activity and social interactions. A restriction on your daily routine, no matter how justified, can make your existence less fulfilling and meaningful as well as increase your chances of fatigue and falls. This is another reason to start working on your balance problems.

Balance issues are likely to worsen as the years pass by. A balance disorder is one of the primary reasons seniors seek medical care. You may feel anxious when you are unable to trust yourself when it comes to balance. Complications from falling can be life-threatening. Falls are the most common cause of injuries—including death—among the elderly.

Exercise can help you prevent falls by reducing several risk factors. Exercise improves balance, stride speed, body strength (especially in the back and legs), cognitive ability, and mood. You should stay healthy and as self-sufficient as you can.

Balance training is essential to strengthen your body and make your muscles stronger for balance. By practicing these exercises, you can cope better with a balance issue like a slip, an unexpected object on the sidewalk, or a trip. The workouts in this book will train and condition your body to adapt better to the task rather than fall.

Chapter 2
BALANCE TESTS

You can't improve your future balance if you don't know your current condition. There are many ways to test whether you are in balance or not. My mind goes to those American sitcoms where you see the suspected motorist performing all sorts of sobriety tests for the suspicious police officer. Some of these tests hold true for seniors with balance issues.

Most seniors will be able to assess whether or not they have balance issues without going to medical personnel to confirm it. What will not be evident is the extent of the issue, as well as whether or not your exercise regime is helping.

These few simple tests can be repeated at intervals to help you assess your progress. It is suggested that you draw up a simple table to capture the date and the result of each exercise. This can be done in a book, or if you are tech savvy in a program like Excel or Word. An example table could look like this:

Date	Exercise	Result
2/8/2022	stand feet together	22 seconds

I suggest you do an initial test to get your baseline, then tests could be done at frequent intervals—for example, every two weeks or once a month, etc. You decide what works best for you.

You should not do these tests unsupervised. First of all, you need someone on hand if you start to wobble; and secondly, measurements and timing are required so it will be difficult to do that without help.

EQUIPMENT

a sturdy chair with armrests if possible

a timer (stopwatch or cell phone)

a helper

A kitchen island or a rail (similar to a ballerina's barre) could be useful, but is not essential.

TESTS

The first 3 tests will be done standing behind the chair. You will use the back of the chair to stabilize yourself before you start the test. It will be there close to you if you start to lose balance. Timing will start once you let go of the chair, and will stop if you grab onto the chair. Each of these tests can be stopped once you have reached 30 seconds. If you need to, you can shake your legs out between the tests.

Instructions for the tests will be given on the page of the respective test.

BALANCE TEST 1

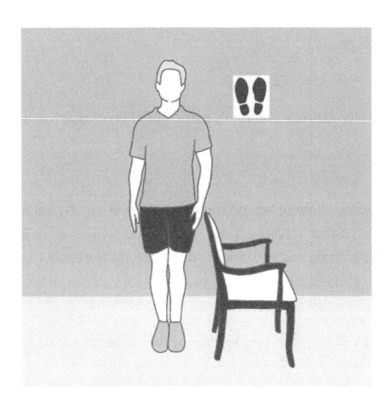

Equipment:

chair, helper, and timer

Directions:

- Stand behind the chair and hold on.

- Bring your feet together. This will decrease the base of your support and will tend to make you less stable.

- As soon as you feel stable, let go of the chair. The timer starts when you let go of the chair.

- You may use your arms to help you stabilize if you wish.

- The timer stops if you grab the chair or you move your feet to accommodate your balance.

Your helper will alert you if you manage to stay balanced for 30 seconds. You have good balance if you manage to reach 30 seconds—well done. Most people on the first time that this test is used will start to wobble and grab for the chair after about 15 seconds, but don't worry if you can't even manage 10 seconds. The exercises in this book will help you tremendously. Remember to jot down the time.

BALANCE TEST 2

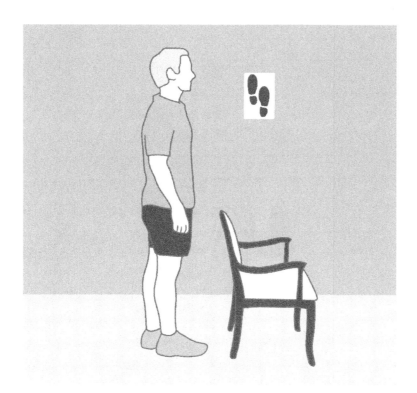

Equipment:

chair, helper, and timer

Directions:

- Stand behind the chair and hold on.

- Tuck the big toe of one foot into the arch of the other foot, both feet facing the chair.

- As soon as you feel stable, let go of the chair. The timer then starts.

- You may use your arms to help you stabilize if you wish.

- The timer stops if you grab the chair or move your feet to accommodate your balance.

Very well done if you managed 30 seconds. Don't stress if you did not. The next time you do the test, you will see a difference. Enter the time on your chart.

BALANCE TEST 3

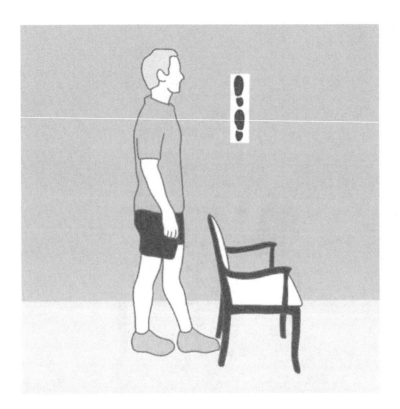

Equipment:

chair, helper, and timer

Directions:

- Stand behind the chair and hold on.

- Place the heel of one foot in front of the toe of the other foot—no spaces and toes to be pointing to the chair.

- As soon as you feel stable, let go of the chair. The timer then starts.

- You may use your arms to help you stabilize if you wish.

The timer stops if you grab the chair or you move your feet to accommodate your balance. This one is a bit harder, so kudos to you if you made 30 seconds. If you struggled more on this one, don't worry. It was hard. But a few weeks down the line, you will be pleased to compare today's time with your fitter time.

FINAL TEST

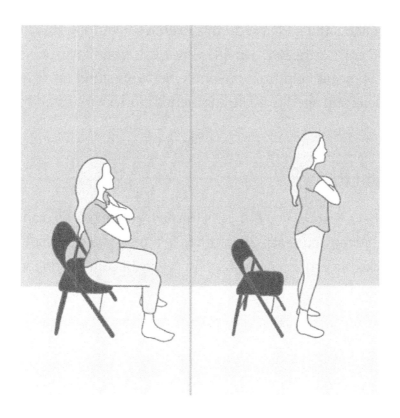

Equipment:

chair, helper, and timer

Directions:

- Sit straight in your chair, feet planted firmly on the floor a bit away from the chair.

- Cross your arms in front of your chest.

- The timer must start as you move to stand up. Try to stand without using your arms to push you up. If you need help to get up, make a note in the table you are keeping.

- You need to stand absolutely straight before you lower yourself into the chair. Do this slowly and mindfully. Do not just thump into the chair.

- As soon as you are seated straight, repeat the exercise four more times.

In a couple of weeks, you will be pleasantly surprised to see how effortless this exercise becomes. Don't forget to record your time.

REMARKS

We stand and sit many times during the day. It's something you do without even thinking. This exercise involves standing and sitting. Please do this exercise mindfully. It will show any weaknesses in the calves, thighs, and core. If these are in any way weak, your balance will be thrown off. If you have to use the armrests or get help from anyone when you stand up, it means that those mentioned body parts are weak and need to be strengthened. You have to stand and sit five times while your helper times you.

FINAL WORD FOR CHAPTER 2

Don't forget to repeat these tests as you progress through your exercise plan. The times for the first 4 tests should increase. When you reach 30 seconds in a test, you can dispense with that test. The last test should get quicker as your core, thighs, and calves become stronger.

Chapter 3

VESTIBULAR REHABILITATION EXERCISES

This is the easiest and most friendly way to start working on balance and dizziness. If the cause of your imbalance has been attributed to vestibular problems, the exercises in this section will help you cope with this condition. When you have this condition, the eyes, ears, and neck are all involved. The exercises have been generated to help those areas.

If there is structural damage to the inner ear, it is unlikely that the condition will heal. All is not lost, however, as our brain learns to handle it. When you are under stress, your dizziness may increase as your brain is too busy helping you cope with the stress. If you have been ill, your brain will be busy helping all of your body parts recover and dizziness will likely increase. Your brain seems to forget that it has to keep you upright. These exercises will help the brain remember that balance is important.

Some of these exercises will disturb your center of balance. It's important to have a sturdy chair close at hand. Walking aids could also be used in some of the exercises, as they help to broaden your support base. A friend or helper will be a welcome addition to your equipment. They will make sure that you don't fall, and will give you more confidence to try the extensions that come with some of the exercises. Other exercises have been designed to get the brain used to sudden changes in position.

If you are using a chair to help you stay upright, then remember not to hang on to it. It is there for support only, and as you get better you can use one hand, then three fingers, down to the tip of one finger as you get more accustomed to these positions.

The exercises are simple to follow. The more you practice, the easier and more stable you will become.

EXERCISES

You will need a sturdy chair and walking aids if you use them. The first few times you do these exercises, you may feel more confident if there is a helper present to catch you if you lose balance.

EXERCISE 1: VESTIBULAR EYE EXERCISE

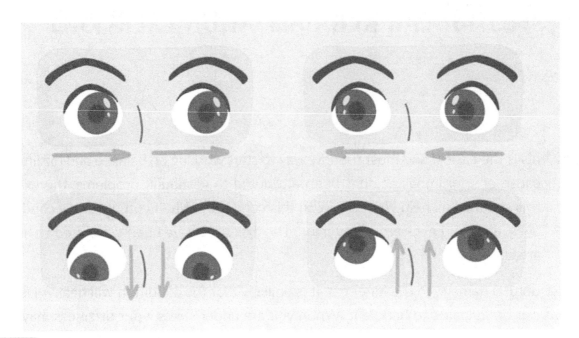

Equipment:

chair

Directions:

- Start with your head facing forward, eyes looking straight ahead.

- Keep your head facing forward throughout this exercise.

- As you breathe in, look toward the right.

- As you breathe out, look toward the left.

- On the next breath in, look up (don't move your head).

- Breathe out as you look down.

Sets:

Do 3 sets and 5 repetitions.

EXERCISE 2: VESTIBULAR HEAD EXERCISE

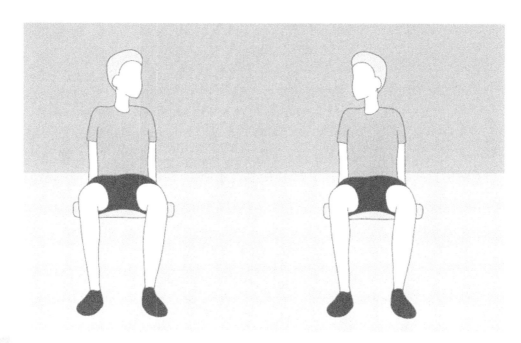

Equipment:

chair

Directions:

- Start by facing forward.

- Turn your head to the right. Let your eyes follow the direction.

- Turn to face forward.

- Turn your head to the left, and let your eyes follow the direction.

- Turn to face forward.

- Tilt your head back, eyes to look at the ceiling.

- Turn to face forward.

- Tilt your head down until your eyes focus on your hands in your lap.

Sets:

Do this 5 times if no dizziness has resulted. Stop as soon as you become disoriented. Repeat this exercise 3 times.

EXERCISE 3: VESTIBULAR HEAD ROTATIONS

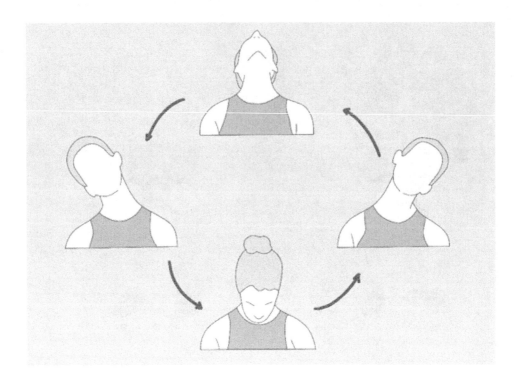

Equipment:

chair

Directions:

- Start with your head tilted back until you feel the stretch.

- Rotate the head clockwise, trying to stretch your neck toward the left shoulder, then to your chest, then to the right shoulder, and then tilt back and bring the head back to the start position.

- Repeat five times or until you are dizzy.

- Rest at this point.

- Then repeat counterclockwise 5 times.

Sets:

Repeat this exercise 3 times. Then, as your dizziness improves, you can do 5 rotations each way.

EXERCISE 4: VESTIBULAR WALKING

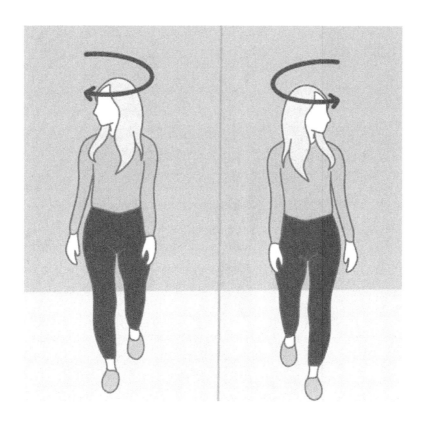

Equipment:

A walking aid is helpful if you use one. A helper will also be useful.

Try to do this exercise in a space that allows you to take about 10 steps forward. As this exercise involves walking, you may use your walking aid. If you do not have a walking aid, a friend may be useful to help you keep on the straight and narrow. They must not hang onto you. They will just be there to stabilize you if needed.

Directions:

- As you move your right foot forward, turn your head to the right.

- As you move your left foot forward, turn your head to the left.

- After about 10 steps, repeat the exercise walking backward.

Sets:

Repeat 3 times with a short break between the sets.

EXERCISE 5: VESTIBULAR TOE TO HEEL WALKING

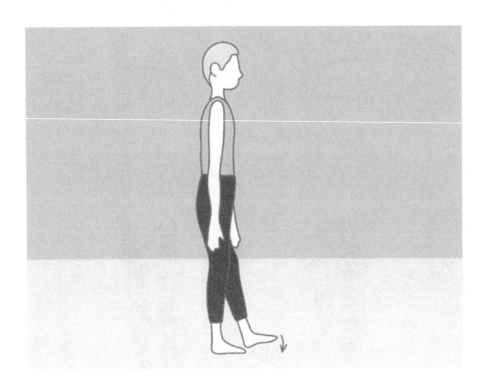

Equipment:

A walking aid is helpful if you use one. A helper will be useful as well.

You can use the same stretch of the floor as for the previous exercise. You can use a walking aid if you need one, and you can ask a friend to help you stay upright. This exercise employs a very narrow support base, so balancing will be difficult. Just do as many steps as you can. You can look down as you position your feet, but that may cause you to overbalance.

Directions:

- Position your feet so that the heel of the right foot touches the toes of the left foot.

- Before you start to walk, concentrate on being balanced.

- Place the left foot so that the heel touches the right foot's toes.

- Continue for as long as is comfortable, or until the designated space runs out.

Sets:

Repeat this exercise 3 times.

EXERCISE 6: VESTIBULAR HEEL AND TOE RAISES

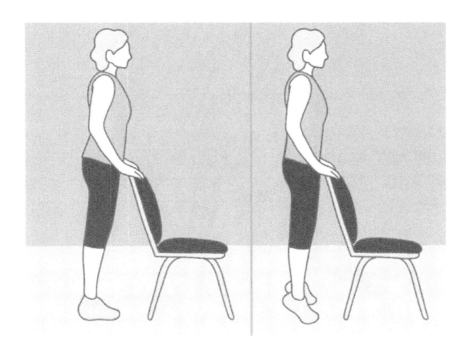

Equipment:

chair

Directions:

- Stand facing the back of the chair, with your feet comfortably (but not tightly) together. Hold onto the chair, but do not grip it tightly. If you are feeling confident, you can release the hold completely.

- Raise your heels just enough so that you are standing on your tiptoes. Don't worry if you can't get too high at first.

- Lower your heels and stabilize yourself.

- Do this at least 10 times.

- Now comes the harder part—raise your toes as high as you can.

- Count to 5, then lower your toes.

- Again, do this at least 10 times.

Sets:

It is best to do 3 sets of this exercise.

EXERCISE 7: VESTIBULAR STANDING ON ONE FOOT

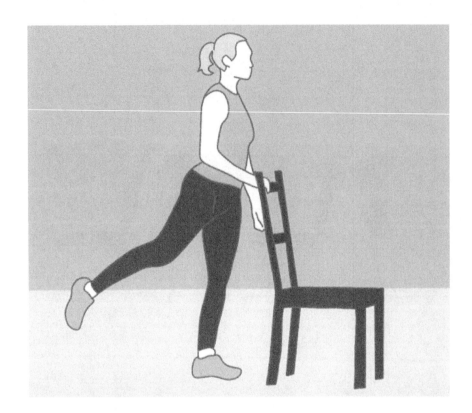

Equipment:

chair

Directions:

- Stand facing the back of your chair with feet in a firm stance—that is, with your feet slightly apart. You can hold (but not grip) the chair.

- Take your right foot backward as high as is comfortable. It will look as if you are about to hop—but don't do that!

- Hold this position for as long as it is comfortable.

- Repeat using your left foot.

Sets:

Do 3 sets of 10 repetitions each.

FINAL WORD FOR CHAPTER 3

With vestibular conditions, the eyes are important. They convey messages to your brain to help it stabilize you. When the eyes are closed, the brain is unable to process the surroundings, and instability results. That is why a lot of the extensions require you to shut off the surroundings or to change your field of vision.

Dizziness can result when your eyes cross your midline. It almost feels as though your eyes develop a sort of shimmer.

As you age, any change in the position of the head needs to be done slowly, together with your eyes and your body. If someone calls you, do not turn your head rapidly toward them, as this will almost certainly cause you to lose balance. Turn your head together with your shoulders and your feet toward the person. This applies even if you use a walking aid.

Chapter 4

SEATED STRETCHES & BALANCE WORKOUTS

This chapter is perfect for those who have a compromised fitness level. If you are still battling with vertigo, these exercises will help you strengthen your arms, legs, and core without the risk of falling. You will need a stable chair, preferably without armrests, as they may get in the way. I like to do these exercises to music with a steady beat, so that I do not have to concentrate on counting. I just do the movements on the beat. The waltz (3/4 timing) or the foxtrot (4/4 timing) are best.

EXERCISES

After vestibular rehab, seated exercises are the easiest to perform for beginners. The aim is to build up to 3 sets of each exercise with 10 repetitions per set. Rest in between each set.

When you are told to hold a position, if not specified otherwise, you can hold for 3 counts or 4 counts, or whatever is comfortable. As you get better, you will be able to hold this position for much longer.

EXERCISE 1: SITTING KNEE LIFTS

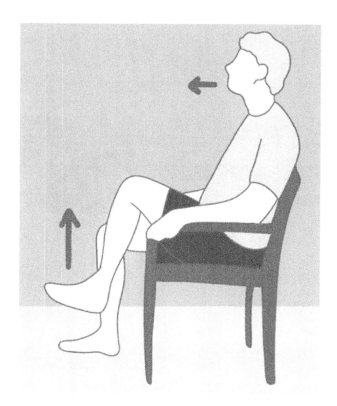

Equipment:

chair

Directions:

- Sit back in your chair with a straight back and feet on the floor.

- Pull your right knee up as high as is comfortable. The object is to touch the chest without leaning forward, keeping the tummy tight.

- Hold this position (You can support yourself with your hands if you wish).

- Slowly lower the right leg.

- Lift the left leg as high as you can and hold the position.

- Slowly lower the left leg.

Sets:

Do 3 sets of 10 repetitions.

EXERCISE 2: SITTING TOUCH THE TOES

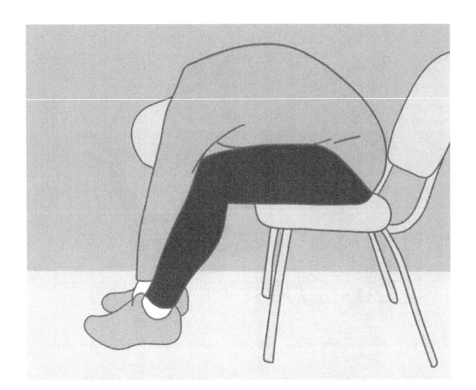

Equipment:

chair

Directions:

- Sit with a straight back in your chair. Move as far back as you can, as you do not want to slip off during this exercise. Position your feet slightly apart.

- Walk your feet forward until your legs are as stretched as they can be.

- Walk your hands down your legs as far as your arms will reach. We are aiming for our toes.

- Hold this position and concentrate on pulling your tummy in.

- Walk your hands back up to your lap.

- Walk your legs back to the start position.

Sets:

Do 3 sets of 10 repetitions.

EXERCISE 3: SITTING HEEL RAISES

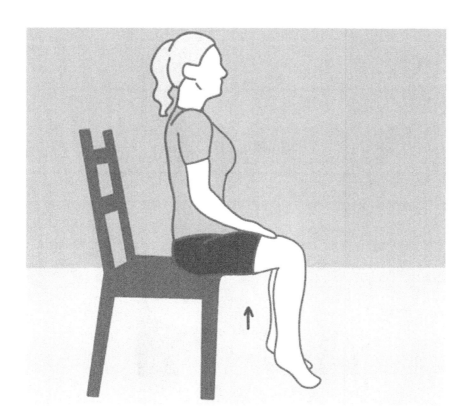

Equipment:

chair

Directions:

- Sit back in your chair. Keep your back straight and your tummy in.

- Position your feet slightly apart.

- Slowly raise your right heel until you are virtually standing on your toes.

- Hold this position.

- Slowly lower the right heel.

- Repeat with the left foot.

Sets:

Repeat the full exercise 10 times before taking a short rest, and then do 2 more sets.

EXERCISE 4: SITTING HIP EXTENSIONS

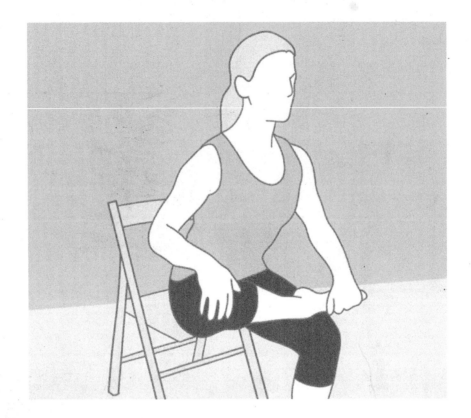

Equipment:

chair

Directions:

- Sit straight up in the chair with your tummy tucked in.

- Lift your right foot onto your left knee.

- Put your hands on your right knee and push down to the count of 3.

- Hold this position for 3.

- Rest for 3.

- Change feet and repeat.

Sets:

Do 3 sets of 10 repetitions.

EXERCISE 5: SITTING SHOULDER ROLLS

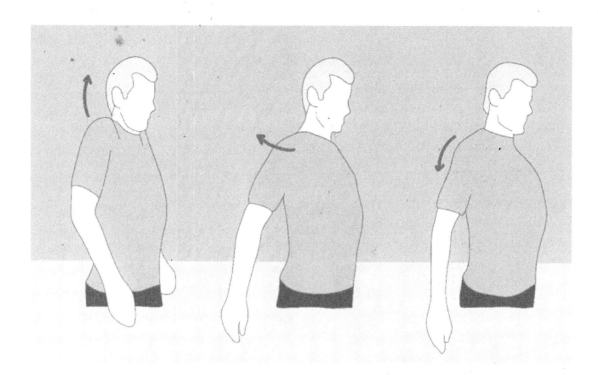

Equipment:

chair

Directions:

You must sit with your back straight and your head up. Imagine a taut string from the top of your head to the ceiling—if you slouch, it will hurt the top of your head or break the string!

- Put your hands on your lap.

- Raise your shoulders to your ears.

- Roll your shoulders back.

- Roll your shoulders down.

- Bring your shoulders forward.

- Then reverse the motion.

Sets:

Do 3 sets of 10 repetitions.

EXERCISE 6: SITTING ABDOMINAL TWIST EXERCISES

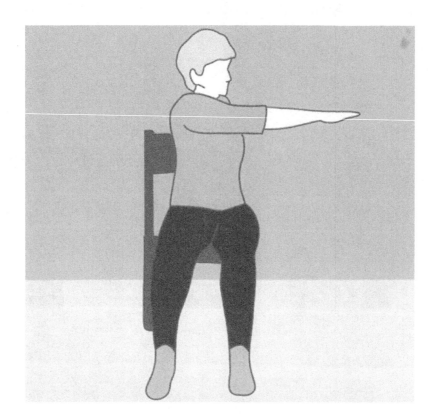

Equipment:

chair

Directions:

- Sit firmly on your chair with your tummy tucked in.

- Raise your arms to the side at shoulder height.

- Look at your right arm and turn your body to the right as far as you can go without lifting your hips, and hold.

- Rotate back to the start.

- Rotate your body to the left and repeat—keep an eye on your left hand and hold.

Sets:

Do 3 sets of 10 repetitions.

EXERCISE 7: SITTING ANKLE CIRCLES

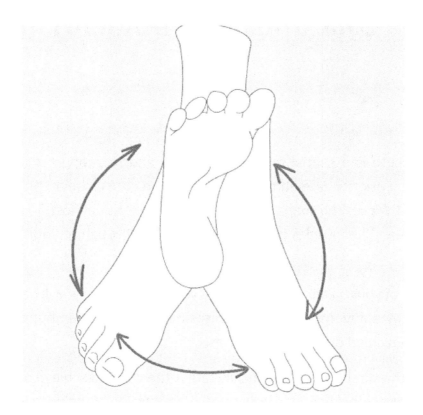

Equipment:

chair

Directions:

- Lift the right foot from the floor as high as it can go.

- Circle your foot from the ankle clockwise 3 times.

- Circle your foot from the ankle counterclockwise 3 times.

- Change feet and repeat.

Sets:

Repeat the whole exercise 10 times for 3 sets.

Chapter 5
CORE STRENGTH WORKOUT

Core strength is essential to ensure stability and to support a person's weight, so it must be a priority. Sometimes we think of the core as being the six-pack, but that is not strictly true. The six-pack is part of your core, but almost 30 muscles make up the entire core. The muscles from your midsection through to your back all make up the core.

The core is the center of your balance. If your core is weak, your balance will be disrupted. Your core will be strengthened by doing many of the exercises mentioned earlier, but only if you keep your tummy pulled in and engaged during the exercises.

This chapter deals with exercises that specifically target the core. To achieve maximum strengthening, you must keep your tummy tight and your upper body straight. It helps to imagine an imaginary, taut rope stretching from your head to the ceiling, pulling your entire upper body up straight.

As you get older, there is a tendency to walk with stooped shoulders. This disrupts the midline and makes the prospect of falling much more of a reality. Try to be conscious of pulling yourself up as straight as you can while walking or sitting. Be mindful of your posture.

Many core exercises require you to lie down on the floor. As you get older, getting up from the floor could be a problem; so the following exercises have been designed to be done sitting or standing. When the exercise requires you to hold a pose, try to increase the time as you become better at it. The holding of the pose is where the main benefit of the exercise lies.

EXERCISES

You need a sturdy chair. Armrests will be helpful in some exercises, but may get in the way for other exercises. Aim to achieve 3 sets of 10 repetitions for each exercise. This will happen with practice. Remember, if you are asked to hold a position, then do it for as long as you can. This will help strengthen the core. Do these exercises slowly and mindfully.

EXERCISE 1: TORSO ROTATIONS

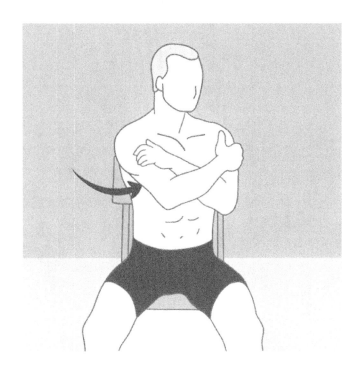

Equipment:

chair

Directions:

- Sitting straight in the chair, give yourself a hug as in the image above.

- Move your hands and shoulders to rotate around the spine pulling as far as you can to the right side. Keep your full bottom on the chair.

- Hold this position.

- Move back to the center.

- Do the same to the left side.

- Come back to the center.

Sets:

Repeat this exercise 10 times. Have a short break, and then do 2 more sets. You will find that your rotations will increase as you get fitter

EXERCISE 2: CHAIR SIT-UPS

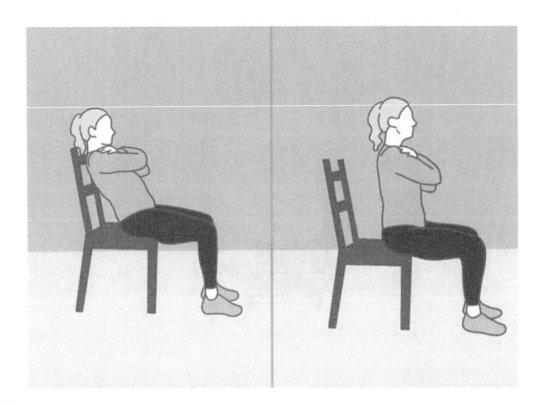

Equipment:

chair

Directions:

- Sit on the edge of your seat and lean back as far as you can, keeping your back straight and tummy pulled in. Be careful not to slip off the chair.

- Using your tummy muscles, pull yourself up to a sitting position.

- Slowly lower yourself back to the starting position. Your tummy must control this movement, so do not just collapse back.

Sets:

Do 3 sets of 10 repetitions each.

EXERCISE 3: SITTING CRUNCHES

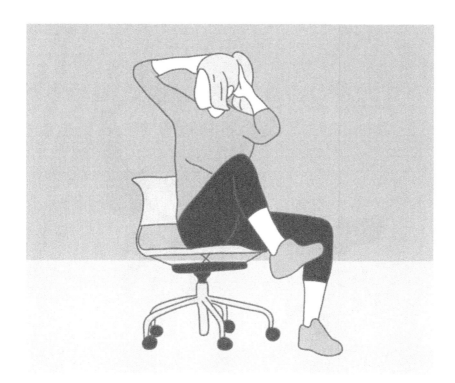

Equipment:

chair

Directions:

- Sit straight up in your chair and cross your arms in front of you so that each hand grasps a shoulder.

- With your feet on the floor, positioned slightly apart, touch the right elbow to the left knee (or as far as you can go).

- Hold this position.

- Straighten up and touch the left elbow to the right knee.

- Hold this position.

- Sit straight up again.

Sets:

Do 3 sets of 10 repetitions.

EXERCISE 4: SITTING LEG LIFTS

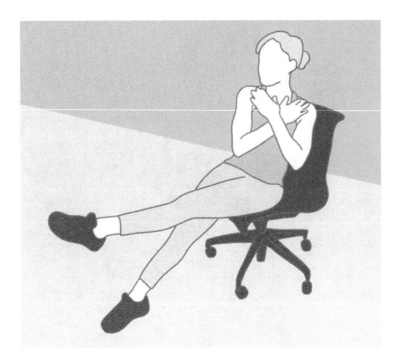

Equipment:

chair

Directions:

- Lean back on the edge of your chair, keeping your tummy tight and back straight. Be careful not to slip off.

- Extend your legs out in front of you.

- Lift your right leg up as high as you can. Use the tummy muscles to do this.

- Hold this position.

- Lower the right leg slowly.

- Lift the left leg up as high as you can.

- Hold this position.

- Lower the left leg with control.

Sets:

Do 3 sets of 10 repetitions.

EXERCISE 5: SITTING BICYCLE CRUNCHES

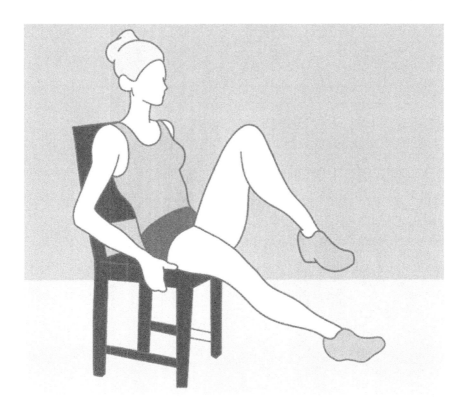

Equipment:

chair

Directions:

- You may need to use your arms to help you at first. If you do, grip the chair or armrests as lightly as you can.

- Sit straight up, tummy in, and raise your legs as high as you can.

- Imagine you are pedaling a bicycle in the air.

- Do as many cycling movements as you can.

If you find this exercise difficult, start by just raising your legs and doing a dog paddle with them. (Think of the children who are learning to swim. They hold on to the side and kick their legs.)

Sets:

Do 3 sets of 10 repetitions.

EXERCISE 6: SITTING SIDE BENDS

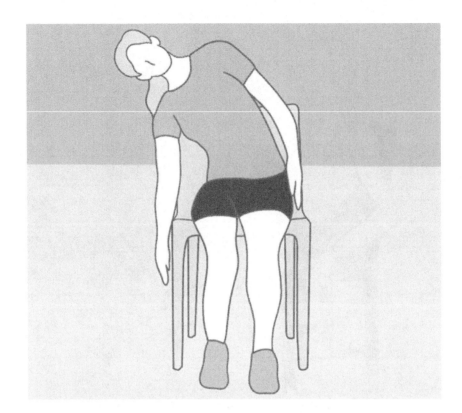

Equipment:

chair

Directions:

This exercise could be done sitting or standing:

- Hold yourself straight and pull your tummy in.

- Bending sideways from the waist, and drop your right arm down toward the floor. If you are sitting, make sure your buttocks do not lift off the chair.

- Hold this position.

- Bring your right shoulder up, hold yourself straight, and pull your tummy in.

- Repeat this exercise using the left arm.

Sets:

Do 3 sets of 10 repetitions each.

EXERCISE 7: BIRD DOG

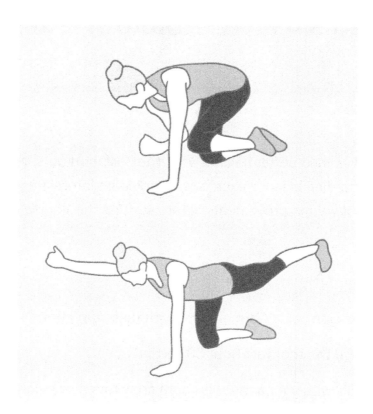

Equipment:

mat

Directions:

- Start by getting on all fours. Then, simultaneously, bring the right elbow and left knee to each other until they touch.

- At this point, extend both in the opposite direction as in the figure above.

- Using the momentum, repeat the movement 7 more times.

- Do the same on the other side.

- Rest 30 seconds, then repeat the exercise one more time.

Sets:

Do 3 sets on each side.

Chapter 6
STANDING BALANCE WORKOUT – BEGINNER

After having gained better balance with the past workouts, you can now step up and perform standing balance exercises. It would be interesting to do the tests again to take note of your improvements before starting this course of exercises.

Never start an exercise session cold. Warm up first with these directions:

- You can do marching on the spot for about 30 seconds.

- You can make windmills with your arms, with both arms together going forward and then backward.

- Or, you could walk for about a minute.

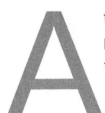 EXERCISES

Please keep a sturdy chair handy for support when needed. A walking stick could help you stabilize as well. You can use the chair to help you balance. Do not grip it or allow it to compromise your posture. You are using it to maintain balance, not to support your entire body. As you progress, cut the support down to one hand, then three fingers, etc., until all you need is the tip of one finger before letting go completely.

With the leg exercises, you will probably find that one leg is easier than the other. As you get better, you may want to introduce weights on your ankles. As discussed in Chapter 5, there is no need to buy weights; you can use household items strapped to your ankles like a book or a rolled up towel.

These exercises must be done mindfully. Concentrate on balancing and doing the exercises as fully as you can. Don't allow yourself to become distracted during the exercises—phones off!

EXERCISE 1: ONE-LEG BALANCE

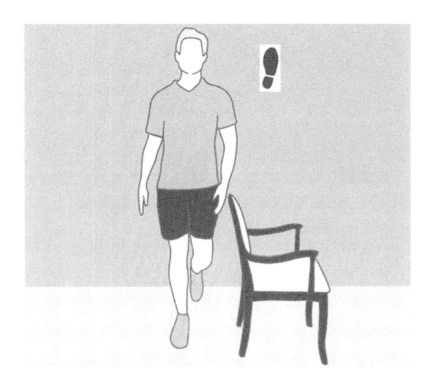

Equipment:

chair, ankle weights (optional)

Directions:

- Stand behind the chair, and hold on as necessary.

- Lift one bent leg up toward your bottom. Try to get the calf parallel to the floor. As you get better, this will become easier.

- Try to hold this position for 20 seconds.

- Lower the leg and lift the other one.

- Try to hold this position for 20 seconds.

Increase the time that you hold the position. Remember, holding helps develop strength and balance.

Sets:

Do 3 sets of 10 repetitions each.

EXERCISE 2: SIDE LEG EXTENSIONS

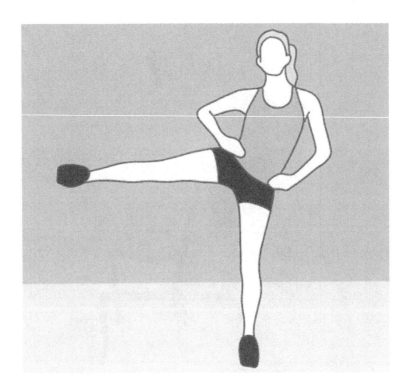

Equipment:

chair, ankle weights (optional)

Directions:

- Stand behind the chair, holding on as necessary.

- Keep your toes facing forward and your body up straight.

- Lift your right leg to the side as high as you can go. Don't collapse your body.

- Hold as long as it is comfortable, but aim for 10 seconds. You can increase the time as your strength builds up.

- Lower the right leg with control. Do not collapse.

- Repeat this 10 times.

- Repeat with the left leg.

Sets:

Do 3 sets.

EXERCISE 3: BACK LEG EXTENSIONS

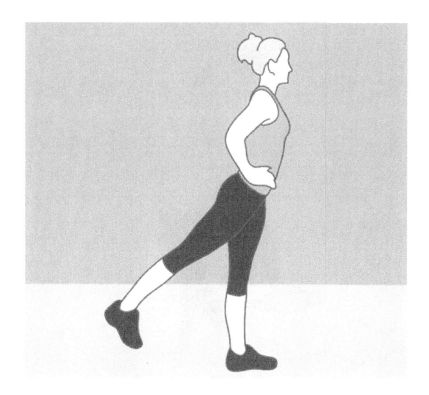

Equipment:

chair, ankle weights (optional)

Directions:

- Stand behind the chair, holding on as necessary.

- Extend your right leg behind you, with your toes on the floor, and reach back as far as you can while keeping your posture firm and upright.

- Repeat this 10 times.

- Repeat with the left leg.

Sets:

Do 3 sets.

EXERCISE 4: ARM-LEG COORDINATION

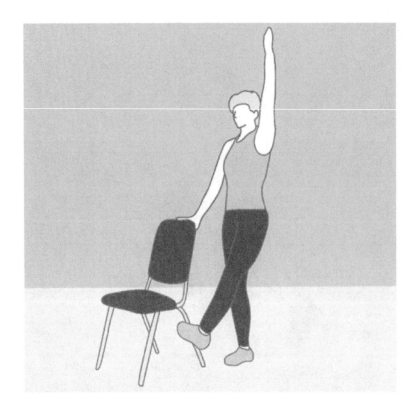

Equipment:

chair, ankle or wrist weights (optional)

Directions:

- Stand behind the chair, position your feet together and place your arms at your sides. You may use the chair if you need support.

- Play the child in class by lifting your right arm up, and stretching it as high as you can.

- Raise your right foot as high to the side as you can.

- Hold this position.

- Lower your right arm and right leg.

- Repeat this exercise with your left arm and left leg.

Sets

Repeat this exercise 10 times. Do 3 sets, with a short break between sets.

EXERCISE 5: TOE TAPS ON A STEP

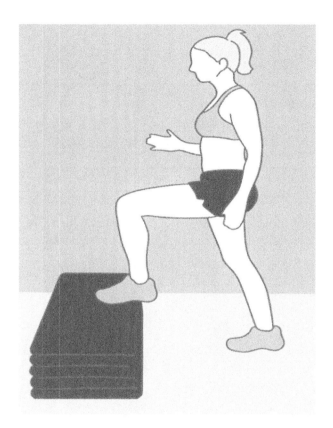

Equipment:

step, ankle weights (optional)

Directions:

- Stand with feet slightly apart.

- Lift the right foot to tap the step.

- Bring your right foot back to the floor in the starting position.

- Repeat this 20 times.

- Repeat the whole exercise with the left foot.

Sets:

Do 3 sets of this exercise.

EXERCISE 6: PENDULUM

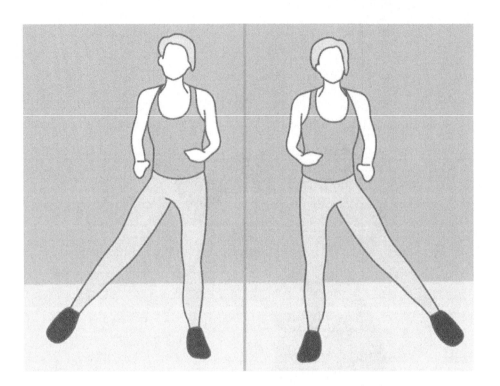

Equipment:

chair, ankle weights (optional)

Directions:

For this exercise, you are going to mimic a pendulum! Your movements must be smooth and continuous, while keeping your posture upright and tummy tucked in:

- Stand behind the chair so that it is there for your support if necessary. Remain upright with your tummy tucked in.

- Lift your right foot smoothly to the side—do not collapse your body.

- Return to the start position.

- Immediately lift your left foot to the side.

- Return to the start position.

Sets:

Repeat this exercise 15 times. Take a break and then do 2 more sets.

EXERCISE 7: STANDING SIDE BENDS

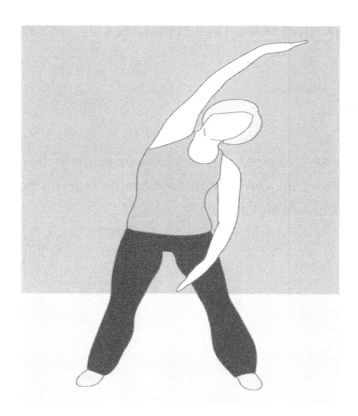

Equipment:

chair, wrist weights (optional)

Directions:

- Stand with legs open wide.

- Extend your right arm over your head. At the same time, lean your torso to the left side.

- Hold this position for 10 seconds.

- Do the same for the other side. Repeat 3 more times for each side.

Sets:

Do 3 sets.

Chapter 7

STANDING BALANCE WORKOUT — INTERMEDIATE

I f you are confident and well balanced after doing the exercises in the previous section, then you will be ready to step things up. Don't forget to warm up before starting. As the exercises get more advanced, warm-ups are important.

EXERCISE 1: BODY FLEXORS

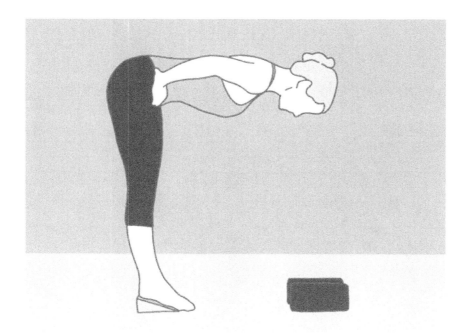

Equipment:

chair (optional but advised)

Directions:

- Stand with feet slightly apart.

- Bend your body forward from your waist as far as is comfortable. Hold the position for a few seconds, then stand uprght.

- Bend back from your waist. Stop as soon as you feel your back muscles being engaged. Hold the position for a few seconds, then stand uprght.

- Swing your body from the waist to the right using your side muscles. Do not let your arms help by supplying momentum. Do this for a few seconds, then stand uprght.

- Swing your body from the waist to the left using your side muscles. Do not let your arms help with momentum. Do this for a few seconds, then stand uprght.

- Repeat this 15 times.

Sets:

Do 3 sets.

EXERCISE 2: BOSU BALANCE

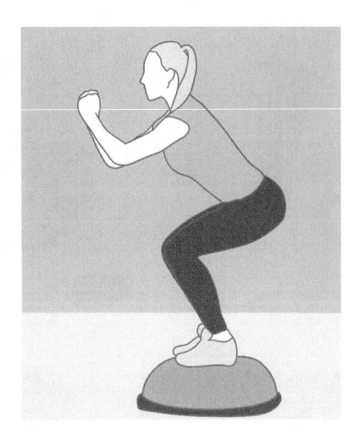

Equipment:

Bosu

Directions:

- Step onto the bosu with feet open wide. You might want a chair or something else to grab onto since this exercise can be tricky for beginners.

- Standing still will cause your feet to move and your torso to contract to find balance. You can increase the difficulty by letting go of the chair, extending your arms upwards, or closing your eyes.

- Bend your knees slightly as if performing a squat.

- Hold the position for 30 to 60 seconds, then rest for 60 seconds.

Sets:

Do 3 sets of 30 to 60 seconds each.

EXERCISE 3: INTERMEDIATE GRAPEVINES

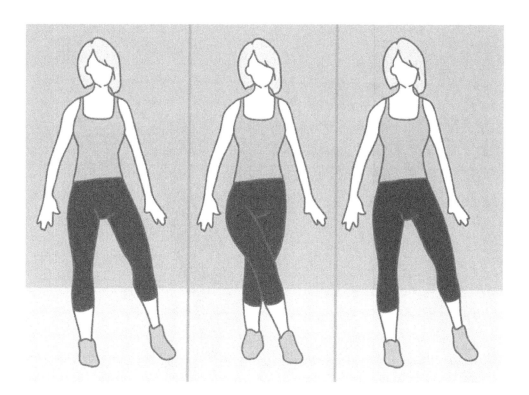

Equipment:

None

Directions:

- With your left foot, step to the side.

- Step with your right foot in front and across your left foot.

- Step your left foot to the side.

- Bring your right foot across, behind the left foot.

- Unwind by stepping to the left with your left foot.

This alternating from the front to the back needs concentration. If you feel a bit wobbly, ask a friend to spot you in case of imbalance.

Sets:

Do 3 sets.

EXERCISE 4: WALL PUSH-UPS

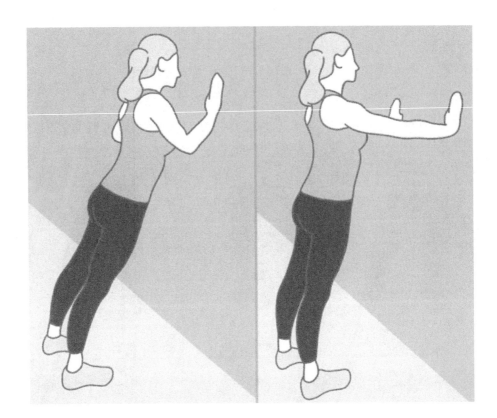

Equipment:

Wall

Directions:

- Place your hands on the wall.

- Keep your body straight as you step back, straightening your arms.

- From your ankles, lean toward the wall. Your forearms should now be flat against the wall.

- Try to touch the wall with your forehead, then straighten up

- Repeat this 15 times.

Sets:

Do 3 sets.

EXERCISE 5: BOSU COMPRESSIONS

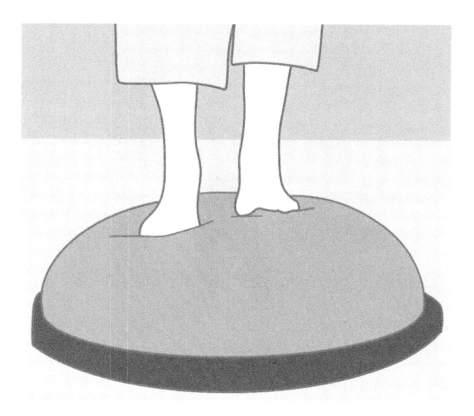

Equipment:

Bosu

Directions:

- Step onto the bosu with feet close to each other. You might want a chair or something else to grab onto since this exercise can be tricky for beginners.

- Once you find your balance, start digging your feet through the bosu one after the other.

Sets:

Repeat this exercise 3 times for 45 seconds each set.

EXERCISE 6: INTERMEDIATE BALANCE WALKING

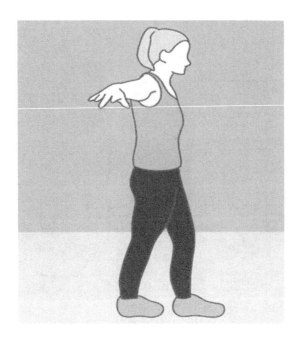

Equipment:

You may need to enlist a friend's help for safety.

Directions:

- Extend your arms straight to the sides (like a tightrope walker).

- Pull in your tummy.

- Take a step with your right foot, but while the foot is suspended in the air just above the floor, hold the position for a few seconds.

- Lower the right foot to the floor.

- Take a step with your left foot, pausing before you put your foot down.

- Take 20 steps, or as many as the floor space allows.

- Turn and walk back.

You may feel a bit like a praying mantis while doing this exercise!

Sets:

Do 3 sets.

EXERCISE 7: SUPPORTED SQUATS

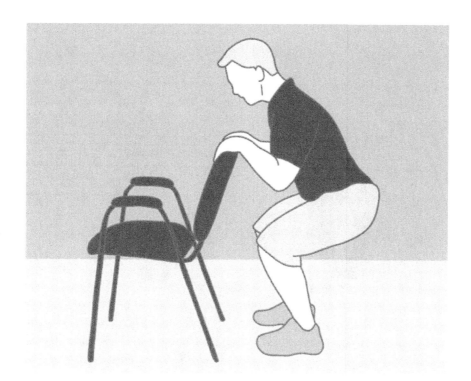

Equipment:

chair

Directions:

- Stand behind the chair, supporting yourself with both hands.

- Place your feet about shoulder-width apart, with toes facing slightly outward.

- Keep your back straight while you squat as low as you can.

- Hold this position.

- Rise up to the starting position.

- Repeat this exercise at least 10 times.

Sets:

Do 3 sets.

EXERCISE 8: TOE AND HEEL WALKS

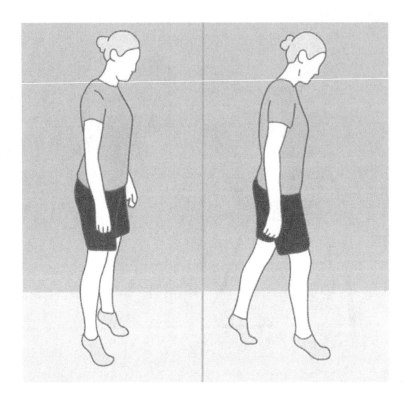

Equipment:

Enlist the help of a friend for this exercise, or use a walking aid if needed.

Directions:

- Remember that tightrope walkers use their arms to help them balance. Be a tightrope walker!

- Walk on your toes as far as your space allows.

- Turn and walk back on your heels. Your toes must not touch the floor.

- Don't compromise your posture while doing this exercise.

Sets:

Repeat this exercise 3 times with a short break in between.

Chapter 8
STANDING BALANCE WORKOUT–ADVANCED

I am so proud you have stuck it out this far. The next group of exercises is going to take you even further along your path to great balance and fitness. By now, you understand that holding a pose is guaranteed to give you a nice firm core that will strengthen your center of gravity. Falls occur when we disrupt our center of gravity. These strength exercises will enhance your chance of avoiding falls.

Even though your balance and fitness have improved, you still need a chair close by. A friend nearby will greatly improve your confidence in some of the exercises as well.

EXERCISE 1: ADVANCED GRAPEVINES

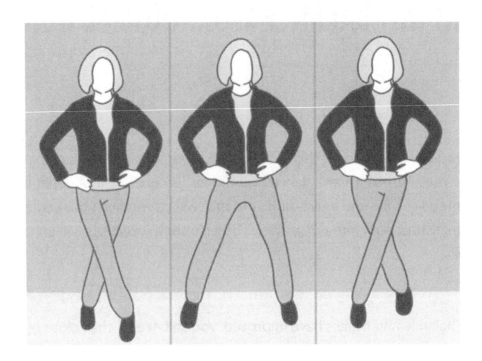

Equipment:

No equipment is needed—but if your balance is a bit rocky, get a friend to stand near.

Directions:

- This exercise is similar to the grapevine in the previous section; but instead of alternating steps to the front and then to the back, these steps are taken in front.

- Step to the right.

- Step your left foot in front and across your right foot.

- Unwind by stepping right again. Try to stay in a straight line as you do this exercise. It might help if you can line up with the floor tiles or the edge of a carpet.

- Continue for 20 steps or until the floor runs out. When you come back, only do the steps on your toes.

- Next, you will do the steps on your heels. Repeat the cycle 5 times.

Sets:

Do 3 sets.

EXERCISE 2: ADVANCED STEP-UPS

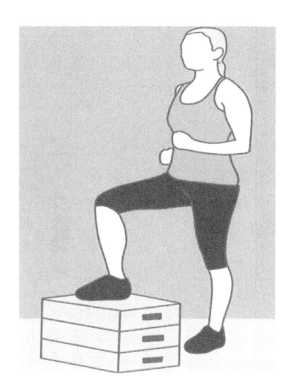

Equipment:

Step/box/staircase

Directions:

- Stand in front of the step.

- Stand with your feet comfortably apart.

- Step up with your right foot.

- Raise your left foot to join your right foot on the step.

- Step down with your right foot.

- Bring your left foot down to the starting position.

- Repeat this exercise at least 10 times.

Sets:

Do 3 sets.

EXERCISE 3: ADVANCED ONE-LEG STAND

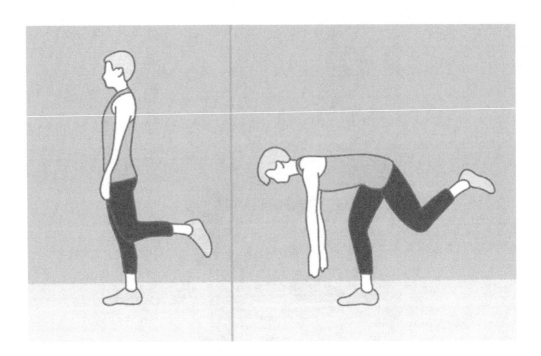

Equipment:

None

Directions:

- Stand behind the chair, and be ready to grab it if necessary.

- Lift one bent leg up toward your bottom. Try to get the calf parallel to the floor. As you get better, this will become easier.

- Now, bend the knee of the supportive leg so that your torso is bending forward.

- Try to reach as close as possible to the floor with your arms stretched down. We aim at least to get the back straight and parallel to the floor.

- Try to hold this position for 15 seconds.

- Lower the leg and return back to your normal stance. Do the same with the other leg.

Gradually increase the time that you hold the position when getting more advanced.

Sets:

Do 2 sets of 5 repetitions each leg.

EXERCISE 4: TREE POSE

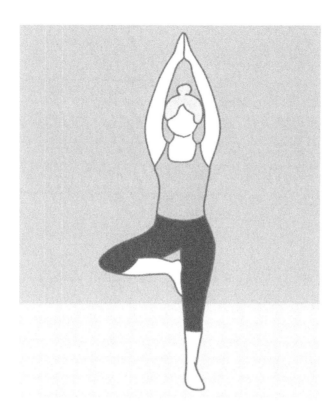

Equipment:

None

Directions:

- Stand and place the sole of your right foot over the knee of your left leg, forming a 90° angle.

- Raise both arms above your head and press your hands together.

- Hold this position for 30 seconds and then switch legs.

- Repeat for a total of two times per side.

Sets:

Repeat this exercise 15 times for 3 sets.

EXERCISE 5: ARM TO LEG RAISES

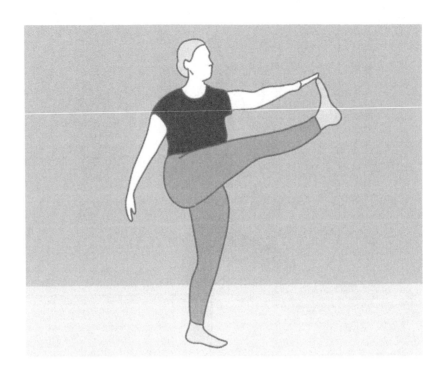

Equipment:

chair

Directions:

- Stand with your feet slightly apart and arms stretched out on either side, close to the chair so you can touch it if you wobble.

- Lift your right leg forward as high as is comfortable.

- Bring your left hand down to try to touch your right leg.

- Pull your left hand up to its starting position.

- Swing your right leg out to the right.

- Hold this position, then return to the starting position.

- Repeat this exercise with your left leg and right arm.

Sets:

Repeat this exercise 10 times for 3 sets.

EXERCISE 6: ADVANCED HEEL RAISES

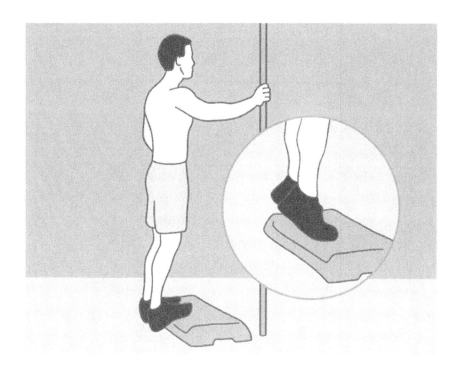

Equipment:

You will need a step and some support for this exercise.

Directions:

- Stand on the step. Your toes and arch should be on the step, and your heels should be hanging.

- Lower your heels as far as you can. You should feel a pull, but no discomfort.

- Bring them up and rise up on your toes as high as you can.

- Lower to the start position.

- Do this exercise with control.

- Repeat this exercise 15 times.

Sets:

Do 3 sets of this exercise.

EXERCISE 7: WALKING LUNGES

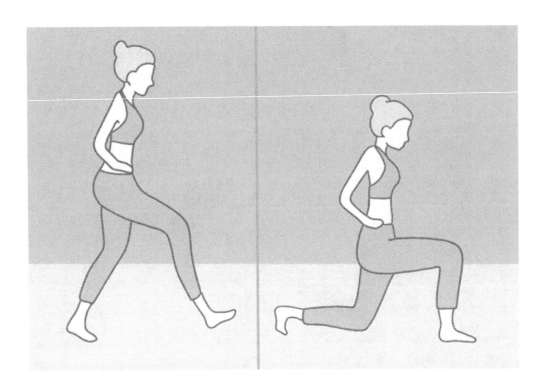

Equipment:

You may feel comfortable to have a friend standing by to help you balance. You will need enough space that will allow you to do at least 6 complete lunges.

Directions:

- Step forward with your right leg, and bend your knee when your foot touches the floor.

- Flex your left knee so that it moves closer to the floor. you will be in a lunge position.

- Hold this position.

- Pull your left leg in to stand up straight.

- Repeat with the opposite leg, stepping forward with your left leg.

- Repeat for 5 steps forward, or until you run out of floor.

Sets:

Do 5 sets.

Chapter 9
FULL-BODY STRENGTH WORKOUT

Balance and strength are related, hence the importance of strength exercises for preventing bad falls. As we age, we need to pay particular attention to our posture. We've all seen those posters illustrating the seven ages of men. In the last age, the profile of the person is stooped. The more you stoop, the more your line of balance is thrown out. This will make the possibility of falling so much more of a reality. When you do these exercises, pay attention to your posture and bring yourself up as far as you can. Make it a habit to be aware of your posture at all times—when you are sitting, standing, or walking.

EXERCISES

Most of these exercises require you to keep a steady rhythm. I find that waltz music helps me keep my movements smooth. Some of these exercises only address posture, while others develop strength and balance. These exercises can be enhanced using weights (remember I explained how to use water bottles in the introduction). Resistance bands can also be used. If you have some firm, thick elastic lying around, loop it to have a homemade resistance band.

EXERCISE 1: BOSU GLUTE BRIDGE

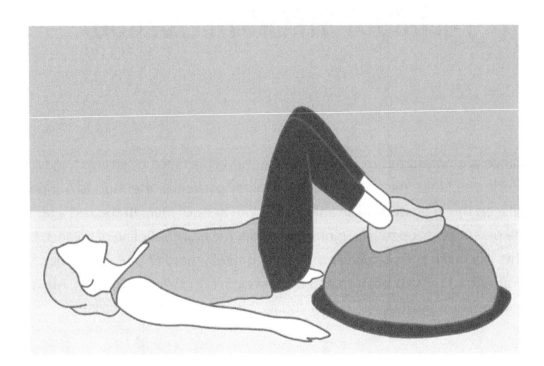

Equipment:

Mat, bosu

Directions:

- Lie down on a mat with the soles of your feet on the bosu.

- Keep your arms along your sides and palms wide open on the floor for better stability.

- Contracts your glutes and lifts your hips as much as possible.

- Hold this position for 30 seconds, then return to the starting position.

- Rest for 30 seconds, then repeat for two more sets.

Sets:

Do 3 sets of 30 seconds.

EXERCISE 2: "W" STRETCH

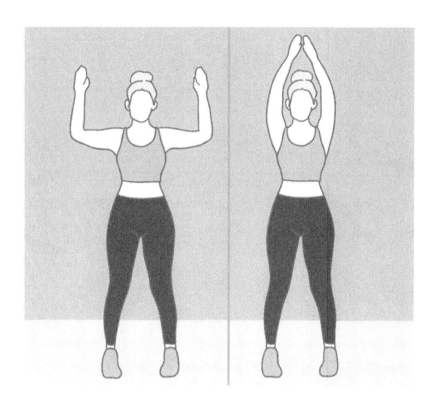

Equipment:

Chair, water bottles.

Directions:

- Stand straight with your feet in a relaxed position close to the chair and your body taut.

- Lift your arms, keeping your elbows bent. From the back, your arms and your head should resemble a W.

- Raise your arms up until they are both stretched above your head and hold the position.

- Return to the start position.

- Do this 15 times.

- If you want to make it harder, hold one water bottle in each hand while performing the exercise. The heavier, the better.

Sets:

Do 3 sets.

EXERCISE 3: FULL-BODY ROTATIONS

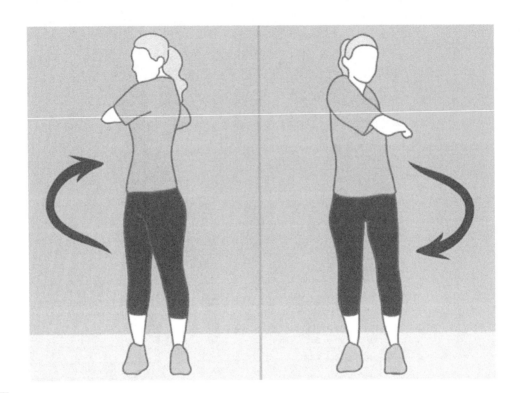

Equipment:

None

Directions:

- Stand with your feet comfortably apart and link your hands across your chest.

- Rotate as far to the right as you can, ensuring you don't strain your back.

- Come back to the center.

- Rotate to the left and repeat.

- Repeat this exercise 10 times.

- Get a good, steady rhythm going.

- If you want to make it harder, hold one water bottle in each hand (close to your chest) while performing the exercise. The heavier, the better.

Sets:

Do 3 sets.

EXERCISE 4: BOSU KICK BACKS

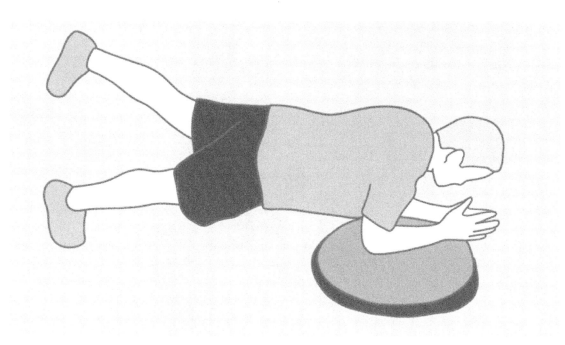

Equipment:

Bosu

Directions:

- On all fours, place your knees on the mat and forearms on the bosu.

- Lift yourself up so that your body is horizontal.

- With the knee slightly bent. Lift the left leg back as much as you can while pressing the heel towards the ceiling. You should feel a nice contraction of the left glute when the heel gets in the highest position.

- Repeat the movement 9 more times.

- Do the same for the other leg, for a total of 3 sets per leg.

Sets:

Do 3 sets of 10 repetitions each side.

EXERCISE 5: BALANCE STANDING

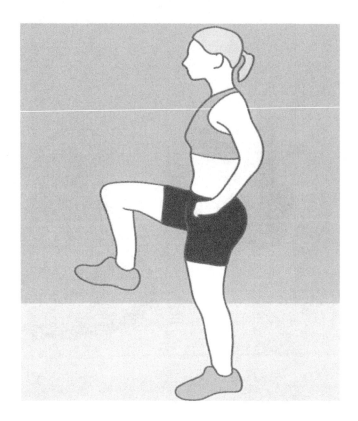

Equipment:

chair

Directions:

- If you need to, you can hold a chair for support. Lift one leg and curl your toes behind the shin.

- Bend the supporting leg, keeping your posture straight and your tummy pulled in.

- Hold this position for the count of 10.

- Change legs to repeat this exercise.

Sets:

Do 3 sets of 10 repetitions.

EXERCISE 6: STANDING BICYCLE CRUNCHES

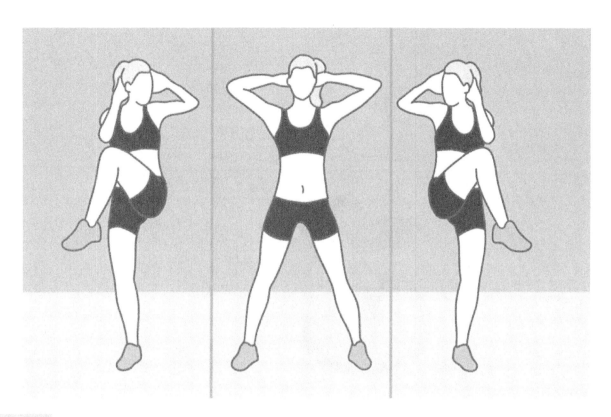

Equipment:

chair

Directions:

- You may place a chair behind you and rest your hand on it for support (only if needed)

- Stand tall with the feet open slightly more than shoulder width and pointing towards the external. Place your hands and arms as shown in the picture above.

- At the same time, raise your left knee across your body as much as you can and lower your right elbow so that it touches the left knee.

- As soon as they touch, get back to the starting position.

- Do the same thing on the other side, and keep alternating until the desired number of reps is reached.

Sets:

Repeat this exercise 10 times per side. Do 3 sets.

EXERCISE 7: BOSU SQUAT

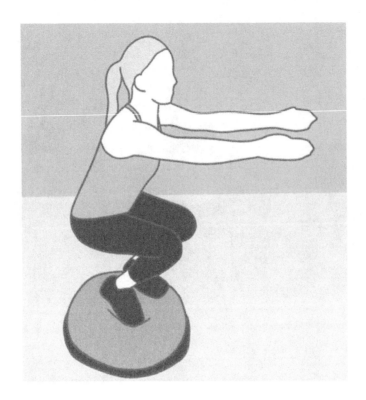

Equipment:

Bosu

Directions:

- Step onto the bosu with feet open wide. You might want a chair or something else to grab onto since this exercise can be tricky for beginners.

- Squat down with your knees bent (pointing outward) as if sitting back on a chair, trying to go as low as you can.

- To help you keep balance, keep your back straight and your torso high, and extend your arms in front of you.

- Come back up, pushing mostly from the heels, not the tip of your feet. You may need to experiment with different foot positions to find one that allows you to retain your balance while squatting. Repeat the exercise 7 more times, for 3 sets total.

Sets:

Do 3 sets of 8 repetitions.

Chapter 10
6-WEEK TRAINING PLAN

Following a smart, well-structured training plan is essential to build balance the quickest and safest way. If you stick to the following plan, you will see improvements after 6 weeks. At the end of this period, do not become a couch potato. Build up a regime that includes an exercise program at least 3 times a week, and go for a walk lasting at least 10 minutes on the other days. If you do not continue with an exercise program, you will soon lose body tone and your balance problems could return.

Just some general notes to keep in mind for your exercise program:

- Dress comfortably and in a way that will not restrict movement.

- Be mindful—none of the exercises need distractions, like reading or watching TV. You can play music though, as it is fun to time your moves to the beat.

- Stay hydrated—have a drink before any exercise, during any short breaks you give yourself, and at the end of the session.

- Warm up before any session. A simple warmup like a short walk or walking on the spot will do. Just remember to move your arms while walking. In this way, your entire body will be ready for action.

- At the end of each week, do the balance tests so that you can make note of your improvement.

PERSONAL BREAKDOWN

Because we are addressing balance as well as getting fit, the exercises involving balance should be done every day for the rest of your life.

WEEK 1

We are going to start by addressing your balance. The exercises for this week are in chapters 3 and 4. I suggest you do the balance exercises 3 times a day—when you get up in the morning, before lunch, and at about 5 p.m. Select which time of day would suit you to spend 10 more minutes on seated exercises for 3 days each week.

The vestibular (or balance) exercises don't require much stamina, but will also help your muscles get ready for the next few weeks. You may need to rest between exercises to regain your equilibrium. Try to only take 30 seconds to rest, otherwise you will lose momentum.

Chapter 4 begins the fitness part of the course, but we will introduce it slowly. Select 3 days to start the fitness course.

TARGET FOR WEEK 1:

- Vestibular exercises from Chapter 3: Do these exercises 3 times daily each day of the week.

- Seated balance workout from Chapter 4: Do these exercises once a day, 3 times a week.

WEEK 2

You are going to carry on with the vestibular exercises from Chapter 3 every day of the week, but you can drop down to twice a day. You are going to include the seated exercises from Chapter 4, as well as start with the core exercises from Chapter 5. These exercises target the neck, back, arms, legs, feet, and almost the entire tummy (which should be pulled in as much as possible). You will have 3 days in the week where you will have to allocate 30 minutes to your exercise program.

TARGET FOR WEEK 2:

- Vestibular exercises from Chapter 3: Do these exercises twice a day, each day of the week.

- Seated balance workout from Chapter 4: Do these exercises once daily, each day of the week.

- Core strength exercises from Chapter 5: Do these exercises once daily, 3 times a week.

WEEK 3

Although the exercises in Chapter 5 are standing exercises, many can be adapted if you are in a wheelchair. Vestibular exercises will be dropped to once a day, but you still need to do them every day. You need to set aside time every day of the week. You will do seated exercises 2 times a week, and standing exercises 3 times a week. You will have 1 day where you will be doing 30 minutes of exercises.

TARGET FOR WEEK 3:

- Vestibular exercises from Chapter 3: Do these exercises once a day, every day of the week.

- Seated balance workout from Chapter 4: Do these exercises twice a week (I suggest Monday and Thursday).

- Core strength workout from Chapter 5: Do the core strength exercises 3 times a week (Tuesday, Friday, and Saturday).

- Standing Balance Workout (Beginner) from Chapter 6: Do these exercises 3 times a week (Wednesday, Friday, and Sunday).

WEEK 4

We now move on to the intermediate standing exercises. You can drop the beginner standing exercises. Your exercise time will be increased to 30 minutes every day. It is best to set aside 30 minutes rather than 3 sets of 10 minutes spread over the day.

TARGET FOR WEEK 4:

- Vestibular exercises from Chapter 3: Do these exercises once a day, every day of the week.

- Seated balance workout from Chapter 4: Do these exercises twice a week (Monday and Thursday).

- Core strength workout from Chapter 5: Do these core strength exercises 3 times a week (Tuesday, Friday, and Saturday).

- Standing Balance Workout (Intermediate) from Chapter 7: Do this set every day.

WEEK 5

The intermediate standing exercises can be dropped, and you can now pick up the advanced standing exercises. It is a good idea to continue the seated exercises, as they will contribute as a warm up.

TARGET FOR WEEK 5:

- Vestibular exercises from Chapter 3: Do these exercises once a day, every day of the week.

- Seated balance workout from Chapter 4: Do these exercises twice a week (Monday and Thursday).

- Core strength workout from Chapter 5: Do the core strength exercises 3 times a week (Tuesday, Friday, and Saturday).

- Standing Balance Workout (Advanced) from Chapter 8: Do this set every day.

WEEK 6

This week you drop the advanced standing exercises, and pick up the full body workout.

TARGET FOR WEEK 6:

- Vestibular exercises from Chapter 3: Do these exercises once a day, every day of the week.

- Seated balance workout from Chapter 4: Do these exercises twice a week (Monday and Thursday).

- Core strength workout from Chapter 5: Do the core strength exercises 3 times a week (Tuesday, Friday, and Saturday).

- Full body workout from Chapter 9: Do this set every day.

FINAL WORD FOR CHAPTER 10

AND AFTERWARD?

Once you have reached your fitness goal, you must not slide back into old habits. Keep up a maintenance program. Set aside 20 minutes per day, and you can follow the suggested outline below:

- Vestibular exercises from Chapter 3: Do these exercises once a day, every day of the week.

- Seated balance workout from Chapter 4: Do these exercises once a week (Monday).

- Core strength workout from Chapter 5: Do the core strength exercises twice a week (Wednesday and Friday).

- Full body workout from Chapter 9: Do this set 3 times a week (Tuesday, Thursday, and Saturday).

Chapter 11
ALPHABETICAL INDEX

This chapter lists all of the exercises in alphabetical order, together with their chapter reference. In this way, you will be able to isolate the exercises that address your particular issue.

Exercise	Description	Chapter
Ankle Circles (Sitting)	Sitting	4
Abdominal Twist (Sitting)	Sitting	4
Arm-Leg Coordination	Standing (Beginner)	6
Arm to Leg Rises	Advanced	8
Back Leg Extensions	Standing (Beginner)	6
Balance (Bosu)	Intermediate	7
Balance Standing	Full Body	9
Bicycle Crunches	Core Strength	5
Bird Dog	Core Strength	5
Body Flexors	Intermediate	7
Chair Sit-ups	Core Strength	5
Compressions (Bosu)	Intermediate	7
Crunches (Sitting)	Core Strength	5
Eye Exercise	Vestibular	3
Glute Bridge (Bosu)	Full Body	9
Grapevines	Advanced	8
Grapevines	Intermediate	7
Head Exercise	Vestibular	3
Head Rotations	Vestibular	3
Heel and Toe Raises	Vestibular	3

Heel Raises	Advanced	8
Heel Raises (Sitting)	Sitting	4
Hip Extensions (Sitting)	Sitting	4
Kick Backs (Bosu)	Full Body	9
Knee Lifts (Sitting)	Sitting	4
Leg Lifts	Core Strength	5
Lunges	Advanced	8
Make a "W"	Full Body	9
One-Leg Balance	Standing (Beginner)	6
Pendulum	Standing (Beginner)	6
Rotations	Core Strength	5
Rotations	Full Body	9
Shoulder Rolls (Sitting)	Sitting	4
Side Bends	Core Strength	5
Side Bends	Standing (Beginner)	6
Side Leg Extensions	Standing (Beginner)	6
Squat (Bosu)	Full Body	9
Standing on One Foot	Vestibular	3
Step-Ups	Advanced	8
Supported Squat	Intermediate	7
Toe Taps on a Step	Standing (Beginner)	6
Toe to Heel Walking	Vestibular	3
Toe and Heel Walks	Intermediate	7
Touch the Toes (Sitting)	Sitting	4
Tree Pose	Advanced	8
Walking	Vestibular	3
Wall Push-Ups	Intermediate	7

CONCLUSION

hope you have enjoyed the journey with me. Life is so much more rewarding in your golden years if you are active. Once you have completed the 6-week plan, don't forget to keep up the good work. You should always be able to snatch 10 or 15 minutes per day to continue with the program. Week 6 can become your continuous session, or you can choose to repeat the exercises at random.

If you are away from home and exercising is difficult, don't make excuses for yourself. Keep on exercising, even if it is a short walk per day or doing some of the exercises in this book. There should be no need for you to abandon all physical exercise. Also, remember to do your balance exercises daily.

If you are ill, then rather abandon all exercise, just rest up. When you are well and have your doctor's clearance, then start with a week of balance exercises followed by the 6-week plan. Remember, no exercise program should be started if your doctor does not agree.

As you work through the exercises, keep music handy—but no books or TV. To make it interesting, experiment with different base surfaces if you have not done so already. A standing exercise will feel very different with different types of footwear. Try slippers, normal shoes, walking, or dance shoes. You will see that your center of balance will change and the exercise will feel different. Standing on a pillow or cushion could disrupt your balance in a good way.

To steal a bit of a phrase from Strictly Come Dancing (James, 2004)—"Keep on toning!"

REFERENCES

Astaire, F. (2002). Pick Yourself Up [Song]. On Fred Astaire - Pick yourself up [Album]. Hallmark Music & Entertainment.

Basic facts about basic facts | Aging & health A-Z. (n.d.). Health in Aging Foundation. https://www.healthinaging.org/a-z-topic/geriatrics/basic-facts

Cronkleton, E. 11 balance exercises for seniors. (2020, May 11). Healthline. https://www.healthline.com/health/exercise-fitness/balance-exercises-for-seniors#exercises-to-try

14 exercises for seniors to improve strength and balance. (n.d.). Philips Lifeline. https://www.lifeline.ca/en/resources/14-exercises-for-seniors-to-improve-strength-and-balance/

Hecht, M. (2019, May 28). 12 stretch and strength moves for ankle mobility. Healthline. https://www.healthline.com/health/ankle-mobility#heel-drop

Home-based dizziness exercises. (n.d.). Vestibular Disorders Association. https://vestibular.org/article/diagnosis-treatment/treatments/home-based-exercise/

Institute of Medicine (US) Division of Health Promotion and Disease Prevention. (1992). Falls in older persons: Risk factors and prevention (Berg, R. L. & Cassells, J.S., Eds.). ncbi.nlm.nih.gov. https://www.ncbi.nlm.nih.gov/books/NBK235613/https://www.ncbi.nlm.nih.gov/books/NBK235613/

Iwasaki, S., & Yamasoba, T. (2015). Dizziness and imbalance in the elderly: Age-related decline in the vestibular system. Aging and Disease, 6(1), 38-47. https://doi.org/10.14336/AD.2014.0128

James, S. (Producer). (2004-Present). Strictly come dancing [TV series]. BBC Studios.

Kernisan, L. (2018, October 23). Why older people fall & how to reduce fall risk. Better Health While Aging. https://betterhealthwhileaging.net/why-aging-adults-fall/

A quote from Confucius. (n.d.). Goodreads. https://www.goodreads.com/quotes/64564-the-man-who-moves-a-mountain-begins-by-carrying-away

10 balance exercises for seniors that you can do at home. (2020, July 17). Snug Safety. https://www.snugsafe.com/all-posts/balance-exercises-for-seniors

The 10 best balance exercises for seniors. (n.d.). More Life Health. https://morelifehealth.com/articles/best-balance-exercises-for-seniors

Vestibular rehabilitation exercises. (2017). Brain & Spine Foundation. https://www.brainand-spine.org.uk/our-publications/our-fact-sheets/vestibular-rehabilitation-exercises/

Your guide to improved balance. (2022, May 26). More Life Health. https://morelifehealth.com/articles/balance-guide

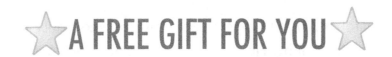

⭐ A FREE GIFT FOR YOU ⭐

Get the audio version for free and listen to the exercises narrated by 65-year old Michael (my dad :D)

DOWNLOAD THE AUDIO VERSION <u>FOR FREE</u>

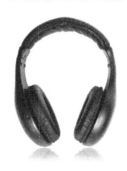

BENEFITS OF LISTENING TO THE AUDIO VERSION

- You don't have to keep the book open!
- You will feel in good company
- It keeps you more motivated

SCAN THE QR CODE INSIDE THE BOOK TO DOWNLOAD IT FOR FREE!

SCAN THE QR CODE BELOW TO ACCESS THE AUDIO FILES

SCAN ME

⭐ HAVE YOU LIKED IT? ⭐

To provide the best quality cases to customers, I would love to hear your thoughts and opinions on this collection.

TO DO SO, I WOULD ENCOURAGE YOU TO

LEAVE A HONEST REVIEW ON AMAZON.

Your comment will ultimately aid me in continually improving my current and future books. I genuinely hope that your experience with my product was positive and memorable!

THANK YOU IN ADVANCE FOR YOUR VALUABLE FEEDBACK

THIS WILL HELP ME A LOT AS A SELF-PUBLISHED AUTHOR!

Made in the USA
Las Vegas, NV
11 September 2023